FOOD *for* THOUGHT

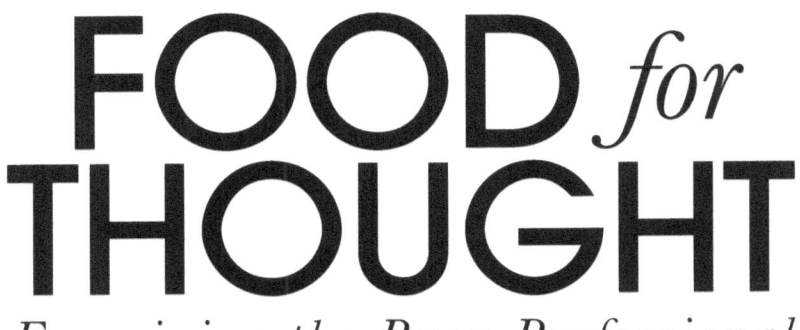

FOOD *for* THOUGHT

Energizing the Busy Professional

STEPHANIE JACK, PH.D.

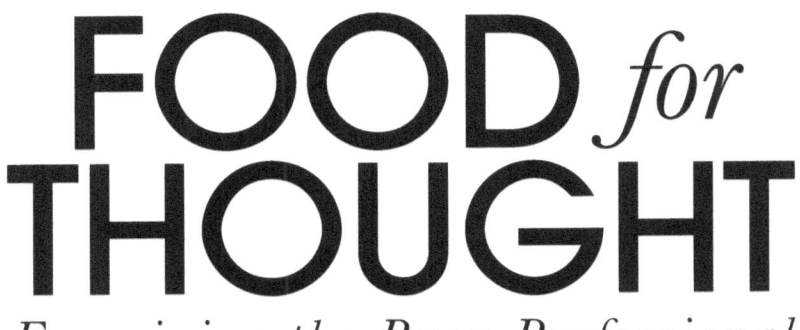
iUniverse®

FOOD FOR THOUGHT
ENERGIZING THE BUSY PROFESSIONAL

iUniverse books may be ordered through booksellers or by contacting:

iUniverse
1663 Liberty Drive
Bloomington, IN 47403
www.iuniverse.com
1-800-Authors (1-800-288-4677)

ISBN: 978-1-4917-8992-6 (sc)
ISBN: 978-1-4917-8991-9 (e)

Library of Congress Control Number: 2016904040

Print information available on the last page.

iUniverse rev. date: 03/04/2016

Contents

Foreword

Professionals are very busy people.

Balancing job, family, home, and children's extracurricular activities in addition to possibly providing elder care leaves little time to prepare nourishing food. Making wise choices in the grocery store isles can be daunting, leading to a grab-and-go mentality. While practical and less time consuming to prepare, prepackaged foods may lead to health problems such as high blood pressure and diabetes.

I have been striving to provide excellent orthopedic care to my patients for more than forty years. Not paying attention to my nutritional needs has placed a drain on my health. The reason for this is that medical school did not teach the value of sound nutrition. The emphasis was placed on building character. Every medical student knows this as "endurance training"—on-call hours on end while in residency followed by building an active clinical practice.

I met Stephanie Jack, PhD, when we worked together in outpatient ambulatory surgery, and she reoriented my thinking. I wondered, *How I can I stay energized throughout the day seeing clinic patients every ten minutes, performing surgical procedures and administrative tasks, and keeping up with scholarly medical and orthopedic journals? When do I have time to eat nourishing food?*

This user's guide is a resource that is easily read. The information is presented at a comfort level that busy professionals can wrap their heads around. The goal of the book is the preservation of overall health through maintaining a proper weight and increasing endurance and vitality. An added benefit to this resource is the educational information on how to avoid wear and tear on the joints and how to reduce the occurrence of degenerative arthritis.

This maverick presentation provides readers with proper scientific information that challenges many supposed truisms that have long needed correction. Stephanie Jack's ideas are certainly worth thinking about.

Peter Van Giesen, MD

Preface

I have been working for more than forty years in various health-related careers as a certified dental assistant and medical assistant and as a teacher. Obtaining my PhD in holistic nutrition was hard work; however, the education I received taught me how to take care of myself and my family.

Shortly after entering the work force as a dental assistant, I developed the habit of drinking coffee. I did not take time to make breakfast, and coffee seemed to fill me up. Occasionally, my car would automatically drive to Krispy Kreme doughnuts on the way to work. I would have a chocolate-iced, custard-filled doughnut (just like boston cream pie!) or a light-as-air, melt-in-your-mouth, warm-right-out-of-the-fryer glazed doughnut. I can still taste them, and that was over thirty years ago. It didn't take long for me to figure out I didn't feel right during the day. Sure, I felt an initial sugar high that I thought was good energy, but I quickly found myself crashing and would have to drink coffee until lunchtime.

Over the years I developed some good eating habits that provided me with energy while I worked a typical eight-to-five job. However, when I started working in an ambulatory surgery center, balancing my nutritional needs became trickier. The day started at six thirty in the morning and ended at five in the evening, which meant I had to get up at a quarter to five. Coffee became the ritual once again. Instead of eating doughnuts, however, I would eat a power-packed breakfast consisting of a hard-boiled egg, a cheese stick, and a handful of almonds—all of this in my car on the way to the surgery center.

By break time I was ready to eat again. Many times I succumbed to a soft drink and a doughnut because the nurses' lounge supplied those temptations in plain sight. And I could not walk by the table without sampling a doughnut. The problem? Soft drinks are liquid candy, (1) and there is sugar in every prepared food (2). When we eat too many foods containing sugar, we are setting ourselves up for disaster. Sugar can cause many health problems, such as migraines, mood swings, and depression (3). Plainly stated, sugar is "pure, white, and deadly" (4).

I wrote this book because professionals are busy people who need to take the time to eat nourishing food. It is stressful trying to balance work, family, and recreation. Choosing nutritious foods is not as difficult as it seems. It just takes a little planning so you can keep readily available good foods like fruit and vegetables, nuts, and real cheese (American cheese doesn't count—it's processed) on hand for snacking.

Ultimately you become what you eat. If you eat healthy foods, take time for exercise, and take time for recreation—and nourish your spirit!—you can reasonably expect to live a healthy life. The book of Genesis states that man was designed to live 120 years. Whether or not you live to be that old in good health with an active mind may be the result of healthful nutrition. This book teaches you how to achieve optimum health for a lifetime.

Acknowledgments

As any author, I must thank a number of people for their personal and professional contributions to making *Food for Thought* a reality.

I would like to thank Dr. Peter Van Giesen, who encouraged me to write this book. The idea came about while we were engaging in conversations between surgery cases. Sometimes we would find out that patients had not stopped taking their blood thinners, which made turning over the operating room a more time-consuming endeavor. During these instances, we discussed the value of vitamins and minerals and how they would benefit surgery patients, especially during postoperative recovery.

Dr. Van Giesen's robust health and cheerful nature impressed me. He told me that taking vitamins and minerals was a part of his daily routine, and he certainly could tell when he had skipped a day or two. Dr. Van Giesen gave me ideas on what supplements he thought would be beneficial for busy professionals who needed to be energized throughout the day while at the same time addressing acute and chronic health issues.

A special thank-you to Tim A. Snyder, journalistic editor and proofreader, who reviewed my manuscript. His expertise helped me avoid embarrassing grammatical errors.

Thank you to Linda Van Giesen for recommending Tim Snyder and for reviewing the manuscript and encouraging me to publish the helpful information in the book.

Thank you to Adela-Adriana Moscu, whose positive statements were inspiring: "Very educational and motivating. The information is inspiring and somehow gently urges one not to only improve one's nutrition but also to reduce stresses, having fun, following dreams and being honest and supportive first of all with themselves and then others."

Thank you to my husband, Terry, who believed in me and encouraged me when I began to lose confidence in myself. He reminded me of my responsibility to share this information so that busy people could choose to live healthier lives.

And thank you to my children, Liz, Maddie, Andrew, and Ana, who daily make wise nutritional choices and whose patience I appreciated while discussing the vegetable de jour around the dinner table!

Introduction

You are what you eat. So the saying goes. If you eat junk foods, such as chips, crackers, cookies, cakes, pies, and doughnuts and drink sodas, it is reasonable to conclude that you are going to get sick. Why? Because depleting the body of vital vitamins and minerals, which exist only in very low levels in highly refined food, almost always contributes to poor biological health and disease (5). In fact, "many diseases can be caused by the wrong balance of essential nutrients in the body" (6).

Sugar, for example, provides an initial high that makes us think they we energized but does not sustain the body with energy needed for long periods of time. It is a good idea to read food labels because you will find out that sugar is an ingredient in every prepared food. Caloric sweeteners like table sugar, honey, molasses, agave, and high-fructose corn syrup are dangerous substances to put in your mouth because they provide empty calories when you should be eating more nutritious foods (7).

Stress is another culprit that can sabotage our health. Almost every major illness can be linked to chronic stress (8). Busy professionals have their fair share of stress. A colleague of mine is a solo medical practitioner. He may experience more stress than a professional who is part of a group because the pressure is entirely on him to pay staff and other business expenses, to take care of administrative tasks, to keep patients walking in the door, and to provide patients with sound medical advice. Compound that with family responsibilities and finding the time for vacation, exercise, and continuing education. I should be shocked to learn that my colleague arises very early in the morning—sometimes at three thirty—to down a pot of coffee before starting his day, but I am not. I am sure he is not the only professional who has habits that can be improved upon. I worked with several surgeons who did not take time to eat lunch between surgery cases. On the other hand, I worked with a pediatric surgeon who took the time to eat a healthy lunch. He was cheerful and a joy to work with in surgery.

Keeping oneself free from disease can be an attainable goal provided the focus is on prevention. Preventing disease by choosing foods that reflect a rainbow of color and regularly taking chemopreventive agents like vitamins and minerals, including antioxidants, will go a long way toward optimum health. These practices are like an insurance policy for your body. For example, vitamin C and vitamin E are synergistic. They work together. Picture a battle going on in your body. Vitamin C is the first line of defense. When that gets wiped out, vitamin E replaces the vitamin C. This strategy is part of an ongoing replacement of essential vitamins.

Exercise is another important ingredient for maintaining a healthy body. It's good to sweat. Sweating releases toxins that can become built up in the tissue in our bodies. Exercise releases endorphins that help balance our moods. I know that if I miss my regular exercise, I am not as pleasant as I can be. One of the receptionists at the gym where I work out said she heard we should work out one minute for every year of our age. She said, "I don't know if this is true." Maybe she was trying to encourage me to work out longer!

As a substitute teacher, I have the opportunity to read essay assignments. One particular writing prompt was on the topic of passion: What are you passionate about? Several students described their passion for exercise. Admittedly, one student wrote that running had been very hard in the beginning but that now she doesn't miss a day. She also said that during a time when she didn't run or exercise, she'd had several bouts of the flu. When she runs daily, she rarely gets sick.

Exercise can be fun. Walk your dog, or dance in your kitchen to music you enjoy. (Or light candles—I use LED candles—on your deck and dance in the moonlight with your significant other!) Swimming, biking, hiking, and even gardening get your muscles moving. I have read that we need thirty minutes to one hour of cardio exercise every day. On the days you lift weights, cut back on your cardio time. It is probably best to consult with your doctor and a trainer for your exercise needs before beginning an exercise program. The reason is to prevent injury and dropout. Also, when you have to be accountable to someone other than yourself—your trainer, for example—the motivation to exercise becomes a daily routine. And you will want to exercise because you will feel so much better when you are finished working out.

Planning time for yourself is just as important as eating healthful foods. One of the benefits I had working in the ambulatory surgery center was a rotating day off each week. Once a month I had a four-day weekend. This was great! I could go on minivacations once a month in addition to taking my regular vacation days. If I planned ahead, I could add a vacation day or two to the once-a-month four-day weekend and have plenty of time for rest and relaxation.

Equally important is nourishing the soul. Whether you attend church services regularly, serve on committees within your church, or go on retreats, taking time to nourish your spirit goes a long way to staying healthy. Taking a stroll along the beach or a hike in the woods where you can turn inward and appreciate nature are also great ways to nourish your soul. A 1990 issue of *Time* magazine reported that heart-surgery patients who had an active spiritual life faired far better post operatively than patients who did not.

Learning to structure meals throughout the day will provide the busy professional with energy. Dr. Elson Haas suggests breaking up the day into seven of what I will call "opportunities to fuel your body." There are four snack times in between three mealtimes (9). For snack times to be beneficial, they should include whole foods such as fruit—not a candy bar or soda. Sodas are liquid candy. One can of soda contains roughly forty grams—ten teaspoons!—of sugar, Studies show that the average person drinks fifty-three gallons of soft drinks per year. And a candy bar such as a Three Musketeers also contains roughly forty grams of sugar (10). Sugar is damaging because it depletes the body of B vitamins, calcium, and copper. It also interferes with the absorption of calcium and magnesium, which are necessary for smooth muscle contractions. This is important for muscles like those in your heart. Sugar truly is pure, white, and deadly (11). The nurses I worked with kept a drawer of candy—chocolate and other kinds. Everyone working in the postanesthesia care unit (PACU) and the operating room helped themselves to the candy. It was addictive because sugary foods produce a heightened release of beta endorphins. Beta endorphins are an opiate-like, pain-blocking brain chemical (12). Stephen Sinatra wrote in his book, *Heart Sense for Women: Your Plan for Natural Prevention and Treatment,* "Eating sugar can be like drinking alcohol. It provides a short-lived high followed by a crash, rebound cravings, and relapse similar to addiction" (13). While fruit contains sugar, the sugar in fruit is not refined. It will provide energy that is healthful, provided it is eaten in moderation. This is important to the busy professional because large quantities of sugar consumed daily will take its toll on the pancreas; long-term consumption could contribute to diabetes.

The message of this book is simple: Professionals don't have to go through life without vitality. They don't have to suffer with disease. And they certainly don't have to succumb to the ill effects of stress. I know that professionals—and anyone!—can feel better by adopting some of the recommendations in this book. It won't take years to see energy and vitality return. In fact, you may be surprised to see health benefits within just a few days.

Chapter 1

What Is Good Health?

How does one define good health? Health may mean different things to different people, with variables in between. Good health to some people could mean taking prescribed medications faithfully and experiencing only minimal side effects. To others it means occasionally taking an over-the-counter pain reliever or anti-inflammatory drug and no prescribed medications. When I worked as a medical assistant, one of my duties was to review medications with patients. Some patients took more than twenty-six prescription medications daily. To these patients, good health was accomplished by these medications.

The World Health Organization defines good health as not only the absence of infirmity and disease but also a state of physical, mental, and social well-being. "Such a definition implies the positive quality of any physical fitness, which means the ability to carry out daily tasks with vigor and alertness, without undue fatigue and with ample reserve to enjoy active leisure pursuits, and the ability to respond to physical and emotional stress without excessive increase in heart rate and blood pressure"(14).

During the 1930s, dentist Dr. Weston Price studied primitive cultures and compared them to their modern counterparts. He discovered that members of the isolated cultures rarely exhibited diseases that were frequently seen in their modern counterparts. The reason was that isolated cultures practiced time-honored traditions by taking advantage of their knowledge of indigenous foods and by taking preventive measures to insure optimum health. Such diets were diverse, some containing seafood, some containing domesticated animals, some containing game, and some containing dairy products. Additionally, some diets contained almost no plant foods

1

while others contained a variety of fruits and vegetables, grains, and legumes. Some diets included mostly cooked foods while others included mostly raw foods. However diverse, these diets shared several underlying characteristics. None contained any refined or devitalized foods such as white sugar and flour, canned foods, pasteurized or skimmed milk, refined and hydrogenated vegetable oils. All diets used animal products of some sort and sea salt. The salt used was not refined or iodized. Celtic gray sea salt, for example, contains many minerals. Preservation methods included drying, salting, and fermenting, all of which preserve and increase the nutritional value of the food (15).

Another factor that impacts health is the quality of the soil where most of the foods we eat are grown. "Unhealthy soil will yield unhealthy plants" (16). This was not an issue until farming became industrialized. Bad farming techniques can cause soil erosion, and growing the same crops year after year in the same soil robs the plants of vital nutrients. Chemical fertilizers and pesticides kill not only bad forms of life in the soil but the good ones as well. Nutritious food for humans cannot be grown in dust. The food industry can also make our food appear and taste delicious, but these engineered foods are nutritionally deficient. Partially exhausted soil that may be rich in most minerals but lacking in calcium will produce foods lacking in calcium. Microminerals can also be affected by poor soil conservation. If the micromineral boron is lacking in the soil, plants equally deficient in boron will be produced. Long-term deprivation of even one micronutrient alters the balance of chemicals vital to health (17).

An issue that should be a concern is the way government officials establish standards that allow certain amounts of contaminants in our food. A report titled "Food Defect Action Levels" (18) revealed what is acceptable. For example, a seven-ounce glass of tomato juice can contain twenty fly maggots. About a pound of macaroni products can have nine rodent hair particles. Frozen broccoli can contain 276 aphids; 3.5 ounces of apple butter may contain five whole insects; and one pound of cocoa beans can contain ten milligrams of rodent feces. The government also allows diseased plants for human consumption. When you think about it, the very foods you eat hoping to keep you healthy may not be fulfilling that role. It's a chain reaction of events. A plant becomes diseased due to poison or a mineral deficiency in the soil. This food is harvested and made available for human consumption. Humans get sick because their human genes become affected from the original poisoning patterns found in the plant (19).

Chapter 2

Disease

The word *disease* is used ubiquitously in medical jargon. One can be diagnosed with heart disease, lung disease, kidney disease, thyroid disease. All body systems can become diseased. Simply stated, disease means dis-ease—not at ease. So when one is diagnosed with a disease, that particular organ or system is not at ease in the body.

Many of my patients state that a newly diagnosed disease is the result of stress. Stress can come from being a caregiver to a terminally ill family member, dealing with a spouse or family member with dementia or Alzheimer's disease, caring for a child diagnosed with cancer, experiencing marital problems or financial problems, living with unfavorable family dynamics, or dealing with employment problems. My patients blame stress for all kinds of health problems. I had a patient in physiatry (pain management) who came in for several epidural steroid injections fairly close together in time. This patient used to come with his wife, but then I didn't see him for almost a year. After that he came often, but I still did not see his wife. Fortunately I got to take care of him before and after surgery. I asked him about his wife. He said, "Oh, she died, and I wasn't with her when she died. I went to the store. I was only gone for twenty minutes." This patient was filled with grief. So I asked him, "Tell me about your wife." He told me she was always taking care of him. Because I had hospice training, I felt comfortable asking him. I learned during my training and from a friend who was a nurse that people often choose the day and time they are going to die. I relayed this information to him. He said, "Do you really think so?" I said I believed this to be true because six months after my dad died, I found a book he had been reading. The passage was dated December 22. Today I took a great leap of faith. My dad died on that date in the evening at 6:05. After recovering this patient from

4

his epidural steroid injection, I never saw him again for a pain management injection. His stress, anxiety, and grief over not being with his wife when she died may have manifested as severe back pain. Once he talked about his grief and found a catharsis, his pain went away.

It may be that some professionals compound their own proclivity to disease because of the duality of their jobs. Health care professionals are trained to respond to "codes." A code could be anything from a red light signaling a patient's need for routine help to a code blue—a patient in need of resuscitation or other immediate medical care. Once I was the unintentional instigator of a group of nurses responding to a code blue. I accidently leaned against the code blue button in the operating room. Wow! Those nurses responded quickly! They raced down the hallway and through the OR doors. I am sure they were relieved there was not a true code. However, what was happening to them physically?

Susan Collins, a family nurse practitioner at North Country Community Health Center in Flagstaff, Arizona, states, "Chronic stress acts on the hypothalamus and then on the pituitary gland, ending in a cascade that causes fluid retention and increased blood glucose. This promotes lipogenesis [the conversion of carbohydrates to fatty acids] in the face and trunk and may be a part of metabolic syndrome and obesity" (20).

Stress can lead to other conditions, such as poor wound healing, worsening diabetes symptoms, irritable bowel syndrome, stomach ulcers, asthma, and autoimmune disorders. Collins states that almost every major illness can be linked to chronic stress.

An early twentieth-century psychologist, Walter B. Cannon, gave a name to stress calling it the fight-or-flight response. A later work by Nobel laureate Hans Selye defined stress as "a chemical or physical disturbance in the cells or tissues produced by a change in the external environment or within the body that requires a response to counteract the disturbance." Long-term stress creates chronic stressors that suppress both cellular and humoral immunity (21).

Joseph Goldberg, MD, reviewed three articles on stress for Web MD. The first article, from the National Institute of Mental Health, was titled "Fact Sheet on Stress." The second, from the American Heart Association, was titled "How Does Stress Affect You?" And the third, from the Mayo Clinic, was titled "Stress: Constant Stress Puts Your Health at Risk." These articles revealed that stress is a normal part of everyday life. How we respond to stress is what determines whether or not we become sick. With that said, stress can be positive, keeping us alert to dangers. But if we become overworked, as many professionals do, stress-related tension builds. Goldberg recommends getting relief from stress. Unrelieved stress can lead to physical symptoms such as headaches, upset stomach, elevated blood pressure, heart problems, diabetes, chest pain, and sleeping problems. Stress, Goldberg states, can also worsen certain diseases. Goldberg also cautions against the use of alcohol, tobacco, and drugs to combat stress because using these products keeps the body stressed rather than relaxed (22).

This statement makes me wonder—is there a correlation between stresses and adrenal fatigue? The adrenal glands, which are located on the tops of the kidneys, make hormones. The adrenal cortex, which is located on the outside of the adrenal gland, produces glucocorticoids, cortisol, and cortisone. Glucocorticoids are increased when the body is stressed. High levels of glucocorticoids in the body contribute to disease resistance and high blood pressure. In addition, the adrenal medulla, which is located at the center of the adrenal gland, produces epinephrine and norepinephrine (23). These hormones are responsible for preparing the body for fight or flight. When the body is confronted with a frightening situation, these hormones increase heart rate and output. They stimulate breathing. And they raise blood pressure by causing vasoconstriction, or constriction of blood vessels (24). It is no wonder that a body under a constant state of stress is distressed!

Goldberg prompts us to consider the following:

- Forty-three percent of all adults suffer adverse health effects from stress.
- Seventy-five to ninety percent of all doctor's office visits are for stress-related ailments and complaints.
- Stress can play a part in problems such as headaches, high blood pressure, heart problems, diabetes, skin conditions, asthma, arthritis, depression, and anxiety.
- The Occupational Safety and Health Administration (OSHA) declare stress a hazard of the work place. Stress costs American industry more than $300 billion annually.
- The lifetime prevalence of an emotional disorder is more than 50 percent, often due to chronic, untreated stress reactions. (25)

The American Institute of Stress lists fifty common signs and symptoms of stress:

1. Headaches, jaw clenching, or pain
2. Gritting, grinding teeth
3. Stuttering or stammering
4. Tremors, trembling of lips and hands
5. Neck ache, back pain, muscle spasms
6. Light headedness, fainting, dizziness
7. Ringing, buzzing, or popping sounds
8. Frequent blushing, sweating
9. Cold, sweaty hands and feet
10. Dry mouth
11. Frequent colds, infections, herpes sores
12. Rashes, itching, hives
13. Unexplained allergy attacks
14. Heartburn, stomach pain, nausea
15. Excess belching, flatulence
16. Constipation, diarrhea, loss of control
17. Difficulty breathing
18. Sudden attacks of life-threatening panic

19. Chest pains, palpitations, rapid pulse
20. Frequent urination
21. Diminished sexual desire or performance
22. Excess anxiety, worry, guilt, nervousness
23. Increased anger, frustration, hostility
24. Depression, frequent or wild mood swings
25. Increased or decreased appetite
26. Insomnia, nightmares, disturbing dreams
27. Difficulty concentrating
28. Trouble learning new information
29. Forgetfulness, disorganization, confusion
30. Difficulty in making decisions
31. Feeling overloaded or overwhelmed
32. Frequent crying spells
33. Feelings of loneliness or worthlessness
34. Little interest in appearance or punctuality
35. Nervous habits, fidgeting, feet tapping
36. Increased frustration, irritability, edginess
37. Overreaction to petty annoyances
38. Increased number of minor accidents
39. Obsessive or compulsive behavior
40. Reduced work efficiency or productivity
41. Use of lies or excuses to cover up poor work
42. Rapid or mumbled speech
43. Excessive defensiveness or suspiciousness
44. Problems in communication
45. Social withdrawal or isolation
46. Constant tiredness, weakness, fatigue
47. Frequent use of over-the-counter drugs
48. Weight gain or loss without diet
49. Increased smoking, alcohol, or drug use
50. Excessive gambling or impulse buying

Additionally, the American Association of Stress states, "Stress can have wide ranging effects on emotions and behavior and on organs and tissues in the body" (26).

Let's consider the disease diabetes. How does stress affect people with diabetes?

The American Diabetes Association states stress can alter blood glucose levels in two ways:

- People under stress may not take good care of themselves. They may drink more alcohol or exercise less. They may forget, or not have time, to check their glucose levels or to plan good meals.
- Stress hormones may also alter blood glucose levels directly. (27)

Mental stress can also have physical effects on the body such as poor wound healing (28).

The Role of Oxidative Stress in Disease

Oxidative stress is damage resulting from an excess production of reactive oxygen species or failure of antioxidant defenses. Antioxidant defenses determine the degree to which one gets sick. During the initial stage of oxidative stress, the body's defenses are mobilized, and levels in the blood and tissues of antioxidant compounds tend to rise. If the oxidative stress is too prolonged or too severe, the antioxidant defenses become overwhelmed because the small molecules like vitamins C and E simply get used up and their levels in the blood decrease. As available antioxidants are consumed without replenishment, cellular damage may occur, leading to the development of disease. Heart disease, stomach cancer, breast cancer, lung cancer, colorectal cancer, and oral cancer are the result of oxidative stress in the body. Diseases of the nervous system are not immune from oxidative stress. Stroke, Alzheimer's disease, Parkinson's disease, motor neuron diseases such as Lou Gehrig's disease or amyotrophic lateral sclerosis (ALS), and Huntington's disease in particular show abnormal chemical changes that were brought about by attack by a reactive oxygen species (29).

Psychological Stress

Some experiments have shown that severe psychological stress in rats leads to severe oxidative stress. One such experiment entailed restraining rats for eight hours. This is something that rats find exceedingly stressful. The oxidative stress is characterized by exhaustion of antioxidant defenses and an elevated level of oxidized fats. The principal damaging agent in this type of stress is the hydroxyl radical that produces stomach ulcers in rats. Such ulcers may be prevented by antioxidants.

It is plausible to conclude that psychological stressors such as long hours in a workplace without sunlight, particularly in winter when one arrives to work in the dark and leaves for home in the dark, could lead to chronic disease and possibly stomach problems of some kind or another. A lack of an opportunity for exercise could exacerbate the condition.

Effects of Strenuous Exercise

Moderate exercise, a low-fat, high-carbohydrate, and high-fiber diet leads to a dramatic decrease in low-density lipoprotein (LDL) and oxidation. It has been shown, however, that extremely strenuous exercise leads to oxidative stress and compensatory rises in antioxidant enzymes and glutathione. This is because extreme exercise leads to muscle ischemia/reperfusion and a greatly increased use of oxygen.

Athletes have higher levels of vitamin E in their red blood cells and vitamin C in their white blood cells than do nonathletes. Sen, as cited by Smythies, has written a good review of this topic. He concluded that physical exercise is protective against oxidative stress in a number of ways. However, overdoing it can be harmful. According to Sen, people's physiological antioxidant status varies widely and thus a periodic assessment of our susceptibility to oxidative stress would be desirable. After a review of the methods that have been used to combat oxidative stress during exercise and their results, he concluded that glutathione is ineffective, probably because it does not get to where it is needed. The antioxidant n-acetyl cysteine (NAC) is converted into glutathione in the body and may be effective. Two test studies were carried out to see whether taking antioxidants actually increases athletic performance. The first, on swimmers, had a negative result. A trial of vitamin E in high-altitude mountaineering showed improved performance at low oxygen levels among athletes. At present we know only that athletes have better antioxidant defenses than nonathletes (30). I worked with two nurses who rarely got sick. I would have to agree that their antioxidant defenses were better than those of most people, because not only was one nurse training for a marathon, but the other incorporated exercise daily into her lifestyle.

Aging

"Whether aging is a disease or not doesn't change our goals, which are healthy disease free aging, the prevention of unhealthy disease ridden aging, prolonging health, and achieving our maximum life span potential." Essentially, successful aging through prolonging good health is the reason that prevention is the best medicine for most of the diseases associated with aging. The process of aging is unavoidable; the combination of the delayed onset of degenerative diseases and aging is not only unnatural and unnecessary but deadly. It robs us of vitality, causes considerable pain and dysfunction, costs much time and money for treatment, and shortens our life span. For the most part, these degenerative delayed-onset diseases are indicators of unhealthy aging effects, not causes. In fact, they are mostly caused by unhealthy lifestyle choices; improper nutrition; chronic exposure to toxic environmental chemicals in our food, water, and air; and the unnecessary overuse of pharmaceutical drugs. The stress of modern life also contributes to the development of many of these diseases. They are largely environmentally induced and do not spontaneously arise during aging. Genetics play a critical role, and heredity is a significant factor in what type of disease we might get (31). However, knowing what chronic or acute diseases your grandparents did or did not have can help you plan for a healthy life.

Chapter 3

Prevention

Arthritis, Rheumatism, and Osteoporosis

Arthritis, rheumatism, and osteoporosis are three of the most common conditions patients present with when seeking treatment. I have taken care of as many as fifty-one patients in one day. Not all patients have chronic disease conditions, and many have extremely good health well into their eighties and nineties. One patient of mine was a ninety-two-year-old woman who took no pharmaceutical prescriptions, had no chronic disease, and took only a multiple vitamin daily. She did, however, have some back pain that was preventing her from doing some of the things she enjoyed. We might ask, how can a person in such good health have back pain?

According to Bernard Jensen, PhD, "Over 50 percent of people in this country have some form of rheumatoid disturbance, ranging from slight pain and stiffness in the morning to the most degenerative stages" (32). Jensen includes osteoporosis (calcium loss from bones) in this category because it is a calcium imbalance problem even though it is not a rheumatoid condition. Millions of people in this country, Jensen states, have these conditions, and diet, exercise, and nutritional supplements could help many of them but not all.

The Mayo Clinic Health Letter (2012), reports that it is not uncommon for most people to experience back pain at some point in their lives. Spinal stenosis is often diagnosed in people aged fifty and over and can be the result of wear and tear of the disks and facet joints. Over time, the facet joints can become enlarged and arthritic, causing pressure on the spinal cord and nerves. Symptoms such as pain and numbness or weakness in the arms and legs as well as other problems are the end result, compromising a person's quality of life.

The Mayo Clinic reports there are many causes of rheumatoid conditions: trauma, fatigue, genetic disposition, sodium deficiency, metabolic disorders, poor food habits, junk food, high-stress jobs or lifestyles, drug side effects, food allergies, chemicalized drinking water, excessive perspiration (sodium loss), glandular imbalance, and excessive use of meat. Many other conditions can also contribute to the development of rheumatoid problems. Bernard Jensen, PhD, believes that 90 percent of patients' aches and pains are reflex pain from some other part of the body. Many of these conditions are treated with drugs. Are drugs the answer? While drugs can offer relief from pain, they don't get at the cause of the problem and they don't offer correction, Jensen states. He believes that the problem with drugs is that they disturb the body's chemistry, cause dangerous side effects, and leave toxic residues in the body. Drugs tend to relieve symptoms without getting at the underlying cause, and although drugs can alter the body chemistry, they cannot rebuild tissue, and they cannot replace old tissue with new, which is what is required for complete healing to take place (33).

Rheumatic conditions generally appear at around age fifty in the majority patients who will get them. In those who do, there is a 20 percent lowered function in all parts of the body due to aging. Waste elimination is slower; thyroid function is lower, which reduces glandular function throughout the body and the lowering of metabolism, which can result in weight issues. In order to take care of arthritis and other rheumatic conditions, Jensen states we need to recognize what is going on in the whole body and take care of everything, including toxic settlements, mineral deficiencies, and compromised immune system function. The holistic approach is to build up the body until the body is strong enough to throw off the problem. We need to understand that every gland, organ, and tissue in the body affects every other part of the body (34).

What Is Rheumatism?

Rheumatism, defined by Bernard Jensen, PhD, is the family of all acute, chronic, and degenerative conditions that involve soreness and stiffness of muscles, pain in joints and related structures. It includes all types of arthritis. Arthritis or joint inflammation can be associated with conditions such as infection, rheumatic fever, colitis, accidents, nerve and metabolic disturbances, glandular imbalances, kidney problems, dietary imbalances (too much meat in the diet), and psoriasis. The basis for rheumatism and all the conditions it includes is a chemical imbalance in the body leading to a local or general acidic condition. Onset of arthritic symptoms may be sudden, but they cannot occur unless body chemistry has been primed. This takes a long time. Osteoporosis does not happen overnight; neither does a slipped disc. These conditions don't come about because of one cup of coffee, one doughnut, or some other kind of junk food. It is an accumulation of these kinds of things that have a cumulative effect that we must recognize. Just as the Cancer Society states it can take twenty years to develop cancer, so can an arthritic condition be triggered by trauma that had already been developing (35). What we must realize, Jensen states, is that anytime we have a symptom of any kind in the body, or any discharge, any pain, any development of a calcium growth like a spur, osteoporosis, a kyphosis (rounding of the back), or a scoliosis, we need to realize it has been coming on for some time.

Osteoarthritis

Osteoarthritis is a chronic disease involving the joints, especially weight-bearing joints. Osteoarthritis is characterized by destruction of articular cartilage, overgrowth of bone with lipping and spurs formation and impaired function. I have often described bone spurs to patients by saying they resemble stalactites and stalagmites found in caverns. Osteoarthritis is the same as degenerative arthritis, degenerative joint disease, or hypertrophic arthritis. Osteoarthritis is more common and less damaging than rheumatoid arthritis. It apparently results from a combination of aging, irritation of the joints, wear, and abrasion (36). There is an extreme amount of acidity in all diseases that bring on these conditions. This comes from overwork, living a tired life, not having enough time to ourselves, not having the proper hobbies to balance the daily routine, and preventing overdoing in one direction, however well intentioned. Often we do not get enough sunshine.

Sodium

Very often we consume too much sodium and the wrong kind of sodium. Many people buy electrolyte-restoring beverages that are very high in sodium, and they consume them on a regular basis instead of drinking water. A friend of mine is a good example of these kinds of people who complain of carrying too much weight. Athletes, whether they are adolescents playing recreational soccer or high-ranking professional basketball players, rely on juices, sweet water drinks, cola drinks, and other types of commercial drinks that can be very high in sodium to replenish fluid as they sweat from exercise. The problem is that these drinks are highly acid producing (37). Eating foods that are high in natural sodium is a much better way to replenish sodium that may be lost through exercise. My son-in-law, a paramedic, repeatedly says that unless you have been vomiting and have become dehydrated because of the vomiting, you don't need to drink Gatorade, Powerade, or any other electrolyte-replenishment product.

I have heard many female patients complain of night sweats while going through menopause. Some have to change their nightgowns and bed sheets due to excessive sweating. What is happening in the body is that excessive sweating carries off the sodium salt that leaves a chemical change in their bodies. When calcium comes into the joints as a result of this change to the joints, a distortion of the spine such as hunchback (dowager's hump) and scoliosis and curvature to the spine may occur (38). These problems almost always result from a lack of balance of sodium in the body. Lifestyle is usually the culprit, bringing on a burning up of the sodium, leaving the body extremely acidic.

In order to replace sodium, eating foods high in natural sodium is best. Citrus fruit and all other fruits and vegetable juices contain sodium. However, according to Jensen these must be fully ripe. If not, they can cause kidney damage in the long run because they stir up body acids and put too much strain on the kidneys.

"The sun is our sodium star" (39). The sun ripens fruit. When it is picked too early, fruit contains excessive amounts of green citric acid instead of sodium. Sodium in nature is sweet to taste. Only a truly ripe fruit is best to put into your body. While you may think you are eating healthfully, eating under-ripe fruits can cause you to develop serious conditions over a long period of time. Degeneration that sets in can cause a hip or knee joint to break down. This is an irreversible condition that requires surgical intervention—total replacement of the joint.

Dr. Fred McDuffie states that the typical person with rheumatoid arthritis faces twenty-three bed days a year plus a higher risk of unemployment and divorce than the national average. People with this kind of arthritis also experience an average seven days a month or eighty-four days a year of restricted activities. While osteoarthritis is not as serious as rheumatoid arthritis, people with osteoarthritis usually spend about fourteen days in bed a year because of joint pain (40).

Each of us is uniquely created; therefore, we can inherit genes from our parents that may predispose us to weaknesses such as lower back problems. But this may not always be the case. Sometimes weak backs can be caused by excess weight. Because people want to lose weight, they start a dieting program that can rob their bodies of the proper amounts of calcium and sodium. What happens next is that the weakness in the back begins to get even more pronounced. As they continue to diet, they take in fewer calories, and this robs the body of the proper chemical elements necessary for balance.

Calcium

"Many people who constantly drink juice should probably have a lot of bio-calcium foods" (41). Many juices are high in sodium, but in truth many are very low in calcium. If we don't get enough calcium, the bones can break down, holes begin to form, and osteoporosis is the result. Osteoporosis consumes the bony material that makes up joints and bones in the body. Calcium spurs can be a result of an addition of calcium to the bony structure. Calcium can lodge in any joint in the body. The lower back is probably one of the places most susceptible to having this problem. Back problems of this type can result from our occupations, whether they involve a lack of exercise or too much exercise. Osteoporosis usually develops in the lower back. People who suffer with arthritis need to have greater amounts of sodium for the joints than the average person takes. They also have to have plentiful amounts of calcium. Many people erroneously think that because calcium spurs have developed and calcifications have formed on their joints, they have too much calcium and that they should not eat more calcium foods. What they really need is to have enough sodium to balance the calcium so it doesn't come out of solution and deposit in the joints. Sodium is chemically necessary to neutralize body acids. It is also stored in the joints and can soften any hard material that may settle in the body in the form of calcium. Sodium keeps the body limber. It is a very important element to have in the body, and it must come naturally from our food (42).

How does one get enough healthful nutrition that contains the right amounts of calcium, sodium, and potassium?

Bernard Jensen, PhD, has one particular cardinal rule worth following. Jensen advocates daily consumption of six vegetables, two fruits, one good starch, and one good protein. Jensen also states that whey is one of the foods highest in sodium content. Making your own menu from the following food lists can help balance potassium, calcium, and sodium in the body.

Foods That Provide Potassium

Almonds	Blackberries	Chicken
Apricots	Blueberries	Chicory
Artichokes	Broccoli	Chives
Bananas	Brussels sprouts	Coconuts

Barley	Carrots	Corn
Beans, lima	Cauliflower	Cucumbers
Beef	Chayote	Currants, black
Beets	Cherries, wild black	Dandelion greens
Beet greens	Chevril	Duck
Eggplant	Lentils	Peanuts
Endive	Lettuce, sea	Pecans
Figs, black mission	Limes	Potato, baked
Grapes	Mangoes	Prunes
Halibut, smoked	Mushrooms	Radish, black
Honey	Mustard greens	Radish, red
Horseradish	Olives	Raisins
Kale	Onions, white	Spinach
Kohlrabi	Parsnips	Turnips
Lamb	Parsley	Watercress
Lemons	Peaches	Zucchini

Foods That Provide Sodium

Butter, cow	Papaya	Squash
Cheese, swiss	Pears	Strawberries
Chinese cabbage	Pineapple	Swiss chard
Leeks	Pomegranate	Veal joint broth
Milk, cow	Pumpkin	Watermelon
Milk, goat	Raspberries	Whey
Okra	Rice, natural brown	

Foods That Provide Calcium

Asparagus	Cauliflower	Dandelion greens
Banana	Cheese, cow, cottage	Endive
Beans, lima	Cheese, goat, cottage	Grapefruit, fresh
Blueberries	Cheese, roquefort	Honey
Bread, whole wheat	Cheese, swiss	Kale
Butter, cow	Chinese cabbage	Kohlrabi
Buttermilk	Chives	Leeks
Brussels sprouts	Cream, cow	Lemons

Carrots	Cucumbers	Lettuce, romaine
Limes	Parsley	Swiss chard
Mangoes	Peaches	Turnips
Milk, cow	Peas, fresh	Turnip leaves
Milk, goat	Pecans	Watercress
Mustard greens	Persimmons	Watermelon
Oranges	Pineapple	Whey
Parsnips	Strawberries	

Know Your Foods

Eating the right foods is not an overnight cure. It will, however, bring on correction over a period of time. Only food can build new tissue. Drugs do not build tissue. Replacing old tissue with new tissue is the way to healthier bodies from the inside out. We might fool ourselves into thinking coffee and doughnuts are breakfast; however, these food items won't build new tissue. New tissue can be rebuilt only with a balanced diet.

"What will correct a disease will often prevent it, and those who have this wisdom to eat right, exercise right and live right seldom have to worry about taking care of disease" (43).

Chapter 4

The Relationship between Health and Diet

Stephanie Beling, MD, writes, "Of all the variables of modern life, diet is one that each individual can directly and entirely control." Beling states that research in and out of the laboratory is confirming an old truth: We are what we eat. And if there is a magic bullet for health, its trajectory goes right through mealtime (44).

Unanimously, the scientific community concurs that changes in the diet can improve a person's health. In fact, the top ten causes of death can be positively affected by an improved diet. The 1990 Dietary Guidelines for Americans specifically recommend a low-fat diet with plenty of vegetables, fruits, and grain products. The Department of Agriculture modified its Food Guide Pyramid in 1993 based on recommendations from a joint Harvard-World Health Organization study, making the base of the pyramid a combination of grains, fruits, vegetables, and legumes. The Food and Drug Administration recommends five servings a day of fruit and vegetables (45).

The media presents, from time to time, headlines proclaiming that certain foods offer health benefits and other foods can affect health. Some headlines advocate giving up red meat, filling up on fiber, and taking pills containing synthetic versions of the latest "health" food. This is just a search for the magic potion, but it will yield only disappointing results (46).

Diets based on deprivation tend to collapse after a short time. After deprivation comes binge eating. When we give up a particular food such as meat for months and then, as a reward, consume meat, the result can be a shock to the system. Consider weight loss. Ninety-five percent of dieters have regained the weight they've lost and have regained it all in five years. Studies show that most short-term weight-loss diets are just as unhealthy as the bad eating habits they try to correct. Bottom line? There is more obesity, there are more problems with our immune systems, and we have not won the war against disease. Deprivation simply does not work.

Forcing yourself to eat just one kind of food such as a carbohydrates or protein cannot compensate for many years of bad eating habits. It is a contradiction in nature to eat just one particular food for weeks on end. This is one of the reasons why Elson Haas, MD, recommends seasonal eating, because it provides the body with a variety of vitamin and mineral sources.

Nutrition in a capsule not only is ineffective but may be dangerous. Take beta carotene for example. During the 1980s beta carotene pills were the rage. After a dozen years, studies demonstrated that they were useless. The supplements had proven completely ineffective in preventing disease and were possibly harmful in some individuals. Instead of taking supplements, experts recommend getting your beta carotene in the form of food. There is simply no alternative to a fundamental change in long-term diet. It is essential for good health (47).

Power Foods

It is not difficult to make the change toward more healthful eating. Power foods are groups of fruits, vegetables, grains, legumes, nuts, and seeds in a variety of colors, tastes, and textures that can be combined in endless ways to make complete meals. Power foods contain substances that may be elixirs of long life and good health.

The key substances in power foods are phytochemicals. These are compounds within plants that have a capacity for reaction and interaction. The nutritional value of plant foods has been observed for some time. Scientific studies confirm that people who eat diets rich in fruits and vegetables live healthier lives.

Starting Point

One of the best ways to tell if you are getting enough power foods is to keep a food diary for a minimum of three days. Be specific and be honest. For example, if you eat a turkey sandwich, list it as two slices of whole grain bread with lettuce, tomato, onion, and mayonnaise. If your sandwich was white bread with more turkey and mayonnaise, list that too. In this way you can see exactly what you are eating. It is helpful to include a Saturday or a Sunday meal in your three-day dairy.

Perhaps your food diary for one day looks like this:

Breakfast:

- cup of coffee with artificial sweetener and powdered creamer
- jelly powdered sugar doughnut

Midmorning:

- cup of coffee with artificial sweetener and powdered creamer
- banana

Lunch:

- Coca Cola soda, 16 oz
- grilled cheese sandwich (two slices of white bread with processed American cheese sprayed with artificial butter product or margarine)
- potato chips

Dinner:

- burger from a fast-food restaurant
- fries
- Coca Cola soda, 16 oz

Snack:

- two scoops of vanilla ice cream with chocolate sauce

How many power foods do you think you consumed? It is probable that the bulk of your meals and drinks contained refined, processed, and chemically engineered foods. Take heart, all is not lost. The following formula can help you begin to eat more healthfully without worrying about calorie counting or gram counting (48).

Formula for healthful nutrition:

- Have one fruit at each meal or snack.
- Have a vegetable at lunch, dinner, and as a snack. For variety remember to include mushrooms, sea vegetables, onions, and garlic along with green, yellow, red, and orange vegetables.
- Eat a whole-grain food or starchy vegetable at every meal.
- Have at least one serving of legumes (all varieties of peas and beans) at lunch and/or dinner.
- Garnish soups, stews, and salads with nuts and seeds or have them in moderation as a snack.

Chapter 5

Balancing Your Blood Sugar

The human body is designed to run on carbohydrates. Protein and fat can also be used for energy. However, carbohydrates are the easiest fuel made for the body. A plant food consists mainly of carbohydrates.

When you eat complex carbohydrates such as whole grains, vegetables, beans, or lentils or simpler carbohydrates such as fruits, the body functions in the way it was designed to do. All the nutrients the body needs are present in these whole foods. These foods also contain a less digestible type of carbohydrate, fiber, which helps keep the digestive system functioning optimally.

Humans are attracted to the taste of carbohydrates, which is sweetness. This attraction to sweetness worked well for early humans because most things found in nature are sweet and not poisonous (49).

As scientists discovered how to extract the sweetness from foods and leave the fiber behind, so began the demise of human health, nutritionally that is.

Sweeteners are a type of food additive, and there are many sweeteners used in processed foods in addition to natural sweet flavor (50). Natural, or nutritional, sweeteners are extracted from real foods; examples are cane sugar, honey, maple syrup, raw sugar, beet sugar, brown sugar, molasses, fructose, corn syrup, barley malt, and rice syrup. Chemical sweeteners such as NutraSweet or Equal are widely used by overweight people (Haas, 1992) or people who do not want to be overweight. However, they are really an opportunity to eat more of the foods that provide the body with fat cells; they really don't contribute to decreasing weight. Being overweight can contribute to diabetes, and it is the sweet flavor we are attracted to in the first place that is causing the entire ruckus.

Natural and Chemical Flavorings

Natural flavorings are simple-to-read-and-pronounce ingredients that are listed on prepared foods. Artificial flavorings usually have chemical-sounding names.

- **Natural Flavorings**: vanilla, kola nut, fenugreek, fennel, licorice, mustard, peppermint, orange oil, cocoa, cassia, anise, ginger, garlic, clove, lemon oil, and other fruit oils.
- **Artificial Flavors**: amyl alcohol, amyl salts, benzaldehyde, benzyl acetate, benzyl alcohol, butyl acetate and salts, diacetyl, ethyl acetate, ethyl butyrate, ethyl formate, formic acid, geraniol, geramyl acids, isoamyl alcohol and acid, linalol, linalyl salts, nonyl alcohol, octyl alcohol and salts, phenethyl alcohol and salts, pinenes, propyl alcohol and salts, rhodinol, salicylaldehyde, and valeric acid.

Note that some chemical artificial flavors can be found naturally in some foods such as fruits or nuts, but most are prepared synthetically.

We may not be aware just how many artificial flavors are ingredients found in foods we eat on a daily basis. Remember—eating one of these foods daily does not pose an immediate problem to our health. It is the accumulation of these artificial products over a period of time that gets us into trouble.

Common Foods That Contain Artificial Flavors:

Alcoholic beverages	Ices	Sauces
Baked goods	Icings	Seasonings
Candy	Jams	Shortenings
Cereals	Jellies	Soda pop
Cordials	Liquors	Soups
Desserts	Maple syrup	Spices

Gelatins	Margarine	Syrups
Gum	Meats	Yogurts
Ice cream	Puddings	

Baked goods can be a huge temptation to busy professionals, especially during coffee breaks. The sugar in the baked goods provides an immediate high followed by a crash. The artificial flavors can be just as detrimental to our health as can sugar, and most prepared foods also contain artificial colorings.

The danger of artificial colors is that they are synthetic and potentially toxic. Artificial colors are chemicals synthesized from petroleum and coal tar products. Many of these chemicals have been used by the food industry as experiments on human beings, and some have been withdrawn because of studies showing toxicity or carcinogenicity (51). We can easily surmise that what we consume in our diets contributes to the degeneration of a modern society. It is no wonder that modern man accepts the aging process as replete with debilitating illness and disease.

My rule of thumb when buying prepared foods, if I buy them at all, is as follows: if you can't read or pronounce the ingredient, don't buy the product—it is probably not healthful.

All forms of concentrated sugar are fast releasing, causing a rapid increase in blood sugar levels. If this sugar is not required by the body immediately, it is put into storage, which eventually becomes fat (52). Refined carbohydrates such as white bread, white rice, or refined cereals have a similar effect to white sugar. The process of refining starts to break down complex carbohydrates into simple carbohydrates. When we eat a simple carbohydrate, we get a rapid increase in blood sugar levels and a surge in energy. The surge is followed by a drop as the body essentially scrambles to balance blood sugar levels. Perhaps consuming a fast-burning carbohydrate with a slower-burning carbohydrate and a protein could provide and sustain energy levels needed for busy professionals. An example could be a fruit such as a small apple, a banana, an orange, or any in-season fruit followed by a whole-grain product such as multigrain bread with tuna, lettuce (a dark-leaf variety such as romaine), and tomato. I particularly like the Healthy Choice entrées such as portabella mushroom with spinach and whole-grain noodles. These can be particularly satisfying.

Because I have a tendency to crash when I don't eat regularly, I have learned to eat every four hours if possible. I start my day with a sandwich made with two slices of thin whole-grain bread and one to two tablespoons of organic peanut butter. The peanut butter does not contain any sugar or hydrogenated oils. At break time, I have a protein, usually scrambled eggs or a plain greek yogurt to which I add my own fruit along with a small handful of raw almonds. Lunch can be a small salad that includes lots of color and a Healthy Choice entrée. Or I bring something from supper the night before. Immediately after work I eat a mozzarella cheese stick with another small handful of almonds. I usually eat supper an hour later. It usually consists of a cooked vegetable, a salad, and another protein. On the rare occasions I snack, my husband and I share an apple.

This menu works for me, but it may not work for everyone. I will add that as I have been losing weight and my blood sugar is more balanced, I have been able to give up the early-morning sandwich. Daily during the week I eat a banana and a string cheese before taking my vitamins. This is working for me as I step down my caloric needs. It is, however, an example of combining fast- and slow-burning carbohydrates with a protein. I try to drink eight to ten glasses of pure water daily. I am not perfect. I enjoy coffee very early just after rising in the morning, and I enjoy a more leisurely cup or two on the weekends. I do drink organic fair-trade coffee, as I believe this is healthiest for the body. Anything that is refined or processed, including chemically decaffeinated coffee, may not be a health benefit.

I do use nutritional supplements such as a multivitamin and individual vitamin supplements, as stress can rob us of vital nutrients. I also use nutritional supplements proactively, given my predisposition for estrogen dominance and diabetes because of familial health history.

Chapter 6

Food Supplements Are Not All the Same

Whole Foods

The buffalo roaming the prairie was a complete food source for Native American peoples.

The buffalo provided the following:

- vitamin A from the kidney, liver, and fatty tissue
- vitamin B complex from liver and muscle meats, including concentrated amounts of thiamin, riboflavin, niacinamide, folic acid, pyridoxine, pantothenic acid, and B12
- vitamin C complex from the adrenals
- vitamin D from sunshine
- vitamin E from organ meats
- vitamin F, all the natural organ fats, including omega-3 and omega-6, and essential polyunsaturated fatty acids
- vitamin K from the liver
- amino acids, proteins from muscle and organ meats
- iron
- nucleic acids (including RNA and DNA) and protomorphogens and cell determinants from organ meats and marrow
- enzymes for digestion and immune function and endocrine support from organs
- amino acids, collagen, calcium, and minerals
- minerals from organ meats

"The buffalo made all this from grass and water" (53). Would these animals grazing on present-day prairie grass provide the same nutrients? Less than fifty years after Justus Von Liebig wrote his landmark book, *Agricultural Chemistry*, which forged the marriage of farming and the chemical industry in 1853, many scientists and doctors spoke out against the poisoning of the food supply (54). Consequently, devitalized and demineralized foods resulted from the following:

- farming methods that do not rejuvenate the soil
- chemical farming techniques that contaminate and sterilize the soil
- refining methods that remove or destroy nutrients from food
- the use of chemical preservatives and artificial colors and flavors that pollute food
- the use of irradiation and genetic alteration that damage the biological structure of food
- the creation of manmade junk "nonfoods" that substitute for healthy foods
- the use of agricultural and industrial toxins that contaminate food through pollution of water, air, and land

Westerners tend to think they have at their disposal healthful foods. They have been tricked by the food industry. Unbeknownst to most people, there are seven deadly fallacies of the Western diet:

1. Chlorinated and fluoridated water is safe to drink.
2. Grains are processed and refined and then fortified with a few synthetic vitamins build a strong body.
3. Animal and dairy fats are dangerous to your heart and vascular systems, *but* synthetic fat such as hydrogenated oil and oleo products such as margarine are healthful.
4. Refined sugar is food.
5. Pasteurized dairy products are a nutritious source of minerals, vitamins, and protein.
6. Vegetables and fruits grown on chemically treated soil are safe and healthy to eat.
7. Animals raised in feed lots and supplemented with hormones and antibiotics are a safe, healthy food source. (55)

This is a far cry from the food available when buffalo fed on pristine prairie grass and pure water, providing whole food nutrition to Native Americans. It is no wonder modern man is riddled with chronic diseases.

Can You Get Everything from Food?

According to author Lori Medford, "There was never a clinical trial proving eating 6-11 servings of carbohydrates would improve the health of the American population." Thinking we can eat better still will not provide optimal nutrition. So the answer is no, you can't get everything from food. Medford further states, "There has never been a study of the American diet proving that we get all the vitamins and minerals we need for optimal health through our food." We can pick up almost any issue of the *American Journal of Clinical Nutrition* and find study after study citing that nutritional deficiencies are linked to heart disease, cancer, and diabetes (56).

Perhaps hundreds of years ago people could get every nutrient their bodies needed from foods. And, yes, it is very possible that Grandma was healthier. I can attest to this fact personally. While I was giving a lecture on nutrition to a group of senior citizens, one attendee said to me, "When I was growing up, we ate meat, we ate eggs, we ate vegetables we grew ourselves, and we ate *lard*!" This individual was celebrating her 103rd birthday. So you see, she probably was much healthier for several reasons. The soil in which her vegetables were grown was not overfarmed and was not fertilized with chemicals. The environment was much safer.

One hundred years ago, we lived in a bucolic era wherein our ancestors took most of their sustenance from the foods they grew, such as fresh fruits, vegetables, and grains. Meat was expensive and in short supply. Most of the crops were fertilized with composted plants and animal manure, and those crops were rotated. These were much simple times. People rarely got cancer. Heart disease was so rare that medical textbooks from the mid to late 1800s failed to include it (57).

So what went wrong, since heart disease and cancer and now diabetes are becoming killers in affluent countries? Such diseases did not occur overnight. Changes in the Western diet have come on gradually over the last one hundred years.

The reason is "progress." Progress is the general advancement of human society and industry over time toward a state of greater civilization. While progress is good, it is also bad. Sir Isaac Newton's third law of physics states that for every action there is an equal and opposite reaction. We can expound on this law, applying the principle to the rise and fall of the health of the American people. This came about through the farming industry. A team of horses could plow several acres for planting in a day. A tractor can plow fifty acres. Fertile soil was turned into a mechanized industry. Oil-based fertilizers and pesticides were employed to boost crop yields. America grew into the largest farming economy in the world. Post–World War II prosperity enabled us to replace time-honored diets. Fat-laden animal products lacking fiber and other critical anticancer agents took the place of fresh fruits and vegetables, and animal products became staples in the American diet (58).

Refinement of food began in the 1800s with the invention of roller mills that were used to process grains. And by the end of the century, the canning industry was blanching food prior to heating it up and sealing it in metal tins. During the 1950s and '60s, refinement of food became more widespread. The TV dinner, which was a highly processed, overcooked meal, could be heated up quickly and consumed from a metal container while watching TV. Processed foods stripped away "unnecessary" fiber, leaving the food devoid of nutrition. To prevent bacteria that could cause spoiling and illness, foods were heated to excessive temperatures, destroying natural anticancer agents and forming potent cancer-producing chemicals. Because these foods were unappealing to the eye, chemists started to develop thousands of food additives. The American food companies were changing the very nature of food's purpose. And people were dying too young from heart disease and cancer. At that time, "few people thought about diet's relationship to disease. Over time cancer and heart disease have tragically become normal parts of life" (59).

"Cancer is a mutiny of your cells." One cell from over fifty trillion cells develops into a cancerous one. This is not an overnight process; rather, it occurs over decades through repeated mutations from toxic chemicals. The cells divide on cue until they are exhausted. At that point the mutinous cell defies the orders that the normal cells obey. Over ten years, the cells become a mass barely perceptible to you (60).

The Importance of Chemopreventive Agents

Toxic substances in our environment, whether they occur naturally or are man made, can cause strain on our natural defenses and elimination channels. Because the human body sustains more than one hundred thousand oxidative hits a day, each cell in turn sustains five thousand mutations. Any one of these mutations could lead to cancer (61). Because these mutations usually do not take place in both genetic strands that make up DNA, this is unlikely. However, it could happen, especially if the DNA is damaged in the same area. Some DNA becomes damaged because we have few natural defenses to protect ourselves from ubiquitous toxic substances in our environment.

A number of systems do protect from the toxic effects of carcinogens. Your cells can repair DNA by scanning the entire length of the strands, then removing and correcting mistakes in DNA. Consuming green tea daily is one way chemoprevention works. Green tea blocks mutagens, is antioxidant, antibacterial, anticancer, antivirus, antipromoter, and antiaging. It reduces allergies and protects against radiation. It lowers blood pressure and blocks nitrosamine formation. Also, eat fresh whole foods that contain plant chemicals to help DNA repair damage caused by toxic substances and thusly help to prevent cancer (61).

What Whole Food Supplements Can't Do

"Whole food supplements can't replace a good, balanced diet and regular meals. They can't replace regular exercise; they can't replace a good attitude" (63).

What should we take? We are unique individuals. Your health care provider may have recommendations based on blood tests, symptom surveys, hair analysis, urine or saliva tests, nutritional tests, or other types of testing.

While I was studying holistic nutrition, I arrived at the conclusion that most healthy people can benefit from individual and combined nutritional supplements. I think everyone can benefit from a multiple vitamin and mineral combination. I recommend whole food supplements because they contain the properties of whole food found in nature.

For the past several years, tests have revealed that I have a slightly elevated fasting glucose level. It has consistently remained the same number every year. I began to suspect my multiple vitamin was causing the problem. I was not taking a whole food supplement. I was taking a supplement two times daily that contained three grams of sugar; this equaled six grams of unwanted sugar. I would caution you to read labels to avoid contributing to elevated blood sugar levels. Another helpful supplement is a good-quality fish oil such as Carlson's. The fish oil is good for your brain and also helps lower LDL cholesterol (the bad guys). And consider an antioxidant complex, one that contains vitamins A, C, E, selenium, and zinc. These work together to help protect your body from unwanted carcinogens that are found in the environment and in processed foods. On Sunday mornings after church, I would prepare a big breakfast. My husband liked bacon, and so did my children. I told them I would make the bacon on one condition. They must eat several orange slices from the big bowl on the breakfast table. Orange juice doesn't count—the vitamin C must come from a whole food.

A calcium supplement is another beneficial supplement. (I take a supplement that contains calcium, magnesium, and zinc.) And a glucosamine chondroitin supplement is good for the joints. I was delighted to find an orthopedic practice in Allentown, Pennsylvania, whose surgeons recommended the same basic five supplements for their patients.

Whole food supplements should be taken with meals. Since they are food, they nourish the body every time you take them (65).

Chapter 7

Physical Activity

Physical activity is needed to improve and prevent or reverse overweight, insulin resistance, and syndrome X (66).

Syndrome X is a disorder that causes premature aging. It causes a sharply increased risk of practically every age-related disorder including obesity, hypertension, nervous system disorders, eye disease, diabetes, cardiovascular disease, cancer, and Alzheimer's disease. Not only does it cause physical symptoms, but it may also cause patients to feel exhausted, spacey, depressed, irritable, or angry when they should not be.

If you are over the age of thirty-five, you may have experienced some of the early signs and symptoms of syndrome X such as feeling sluggish physically and mentally after you eat and at other times, weight gain, having trouble losing weight, and having higher and higher blood pressure readings year after year.

Your cholesterol, triglyceride, and blood sugar levels can also be on the rise. Typically these are symptoms that all too often are accepted as signs of aging, but they can all be reversed (67). "Regular exercise, started as early in life as possible and continued throughout life, helps to maintain a normal or even lower than normal heart rate. This can prevent an early death from cardiovascular disease, prolonging health, and promote longevity. You need to exercise every day, one and one half hours minimum averaging seven to nine hours each week" (68). Dr. Andrew Weil, alternative medicine pioneer, states, "The key to staying young is not to buy into the vision of yourself as an old person. One needs to stay mentally and physically active" (69). Any exercise is beneficial. You don't have to set yourself up for failure thinking that if you can't run, take aerobics or some other structured form of exercise, you are doomed. Increasing physical exercise in any way is beneficial. Try gardening, taking the stairs, dancing with a partner or by yourself, or walking the dog several times a week. Exercise should be fun (70)!

"Everyone should do some exercise every day." Walking in the early morning, and yoga stretching, Lad believes, are good enough for most people, and aerobic exercise may also be helpful (71).

We should not overdo it when it comes to exercise. Exercise should keep the body flexible and limber (72). Our Paleolithic ancestors got their exercise in the form of regular and continuous walking. We believe that they trekked long distances. Also, sprinting during the hunt or retreating from dangerous animals involved short bursts of energy. "A brisk walk is something that almost anyone can do." Swimming is very good, and a brisk walk can be performed by the elderly as well (73).

Modern men and women, particularly in North America, often get their "exercise" by walking to and from the car—the closer to the destination the better—and channel surfing with the TV remote control.

People fall into different categories with regard to exercise:

- weekend warriors who don't exercise during the week but exercise like crazy on the weekends
- reluctant "model" exercisers who hate going to exercise class but will grudgingly follow the recommended guidelines of thirty minutes of aerobic exercise three or more times a week
- runners, weight lifters, and other athletes who engage in vigorous exercise or extreme weight-bearing exercise several times a week
- people who walk a lot and are moderately physically active in other ways throughout the day

The people in the last group follow the Paleolithic model more closely than any other group listed. Physical activity, in the form of walking or gardening for example, may not seem like exercise, but it is! This form of exercise is much better for you in the long run than what most people consider exercise.

There are problems associated with the three other exercise groups. For example: weekend warriors don't exercise at all during the week, so their muscles and cardiovascular systems are out of shape. When they do exercise for several hours on end, they stress their systems and often experience sore muscles for several days. Most people do not realize that weekend warriors are generally out of shape. They are prone to more injuries, and their hearts are out of shape. Overdoing exercise on the weekends stresses the cardiovascular system, and that can lead to a greater likelihood of heart attack. (75).

The reluctant "model" exercisers, who are usually very health conscious and try to do the right thing such as exercise and eat a low-fat, high-carbohydrate diet, have problems such as weight gain even though they seem to be doing everything right. The reason is that they typically dislike what they are doing and pass up other fun activities. Resentment creates rebellion, which in turn causes dropout rates. Those who drop out can become disgusted with themselves and decide not to exercise at all. A second reason this method doesn't work is that "if we ignore our feelings and force ourselves to go to class, we don't get as many benefits as we should from exercise because we don't experience joy in what we are doing" (76).

People who exercise vigorously or engage in extreme weight-bearing exercises several times a week are at high risk for injury because these exercises go against our ancestral nature. Humans did not evolve to run on pavement for miles at a time day after day. And they didn't bench press 150 or more pounds. Instead they walked and carried lighter loads such as young children and ten to thirty pounds of food for longer stretches of time (77). Some people may benefit from these vigorous types of exercise, but not all. For the most positive outcome, it is far more beneficial to replicate the type of exercise our ancestors engaged in daily.

The Benefits of Regular Exercise

The benefits of moderate exercise are many:

- helps the body burn calories to control or lose weight
- builds muscle and increases muscle strength
- lowers body fat
- increases insulin sensitivity (or receptivity) in normal subjects, and insulin resistance in children of diabetic parents and diabetics
- boosts immunity, helping the body fight off illness and disease
- helps build bone density in people under thirty and slows bone loss in older people
- boosts optimism and feelings of well being
- significantly reduces stress, anxiety, and depression
- improves sleep, concentration, and academic or job performance
- lowers blood glucose, cholesterol, and triglyceride levels
- reduces blood pressure
- significantly reduces the risk of cardiovascular disease, type 2 diabetes, and other diseases

Walking is the best form of regular physical exercise because it is evolutionary; we were designed to do it, and it is the best all-around form of physical activity for everyday living (77). Research shows that exercise is beneficial for recovering from cancer. It helps to reduce stress (78). What is exciting about exercising and cancer is that exercise strengthens the body and increases circulation. Laboratory studies show that cancer cells cannot grow in highly oxygenated environments, which prevents the double dividing cells from dividing (79). Another benefit of exercise is the release of endorphins that provide powerful stress relief. Endorphins are natural morphines. People who exercise sleep better; they enter into a deeper level of sleep for longer periods of time (80).

Perhaps the most robust people living during the early twentieth century were discovered in Europe among the isolated Swiss. This community lived high in the Alpine region of the Loetschental Valley (81). Exercise in the form of work appeared to be extremely beneficial to a sixty-two-year-old woman living in this Alpine region. Her task was to carry enormous loads of rye on her back at an altitude of five thousand feet. This woman was extremely "well developed and preserved" (82). How many "modern" sixty-two-year-old women can boast of such physical well-being? While I'm not sixty-two, my goal is to strive to be as healthy as this woman.

Some form of exercise every day is beneficial. While not all of us enjoy exercise, the overall consensus is that brisk walking is well suited to most people. The following lists suggests some rather creative ways of walking:

- Begin your day with a quick walk around the block, or make some time for a stroll during your lunch break. A quick walk does wonders for dealing with work stress. People can experience decreased fatigue and tension for as long as two hours after taking a brisk, ten-minute walk.
- Park your car at a spot farther away from work or the shopping center than you normally do, and walk the extra distance.
- At work, refrain from e-mailing coworkers; rather, walk down the hall or down a floor to deliver messages or exchange information. (It has been calculated that spending two minutes an hour to send coworkers e-mails instead of walking to speak to them, day after day, could result in the gain of eleven pounds of fat over a decade.)
- Walk up and down stairs instead of taking the elevator.
- After work, walk to your mailbox, and walk around the block to relax and walk away any troubles you experience at work.
- Ask a friend to join you for a walk, and then talk with him or her as you walk.
- Ask your friend to go on a short hike with you, take a picnic lunch, and commune with nature.

- Combine a little romance with physical activity by going on regular moonlight walks with a significant other.
- Take your baby for a stroll and point out birds, flowers, animals, and other signs of nature along the way.
- Take your kids for a walk around the zoo.
- Walk your dog as often as you can.
- If a grocery store, convenience store, or drug store is within walking distance of your home, save some gas and get into the habit of walking to do your shopping and carrying your purchases home.
- If the weather is bad outside, drive to a shopping center and walk from end to end.
- If you become bored with the places you regularly walk, take the time to drive yourself somewhere else—a park, a wilderness area, the beach, a downtown cultural area, or an amusement park.
- When vacationing, go to towns that have sightseeing areas or interesting places you can visit on foot. (83)

There are other fun types of physical activity that create variety such as recreational biking, dancing, swimming, gardening, and lawn work. Playing with your kids or grandkids can be fun too. Favorites like hopscotch, kite flying, horseback riding, and sailing are great forms of exercise.

It is also important to have playtime with adults. Dancing is a good social activity. Or try bowling or golfing. If you are able to walk the golf course, it is better than riding in the cart.

Physical activity forces the body to burn more glucose and to use insulin more efficiently. Many people don't have the desire to pursue structured exercises such as jogging, aerobics, or body building, but being physically active as much as possible is important to help prevent insulin resistance, syndrome X, and other chronic degenerative diseases

Chapter 8

Executives and Travel

Executives have, perhaps, lives that are most highly compromised by stress-related issues. Executives typically have very busy lives with many responsibilities, all of which is compounded with travel. Recently, my husband and I had travel plans that involved a 6:00 a.m. flight. This doesn't sound like a big deal. Too me it was very stressful. This meant getting up at one o'clock to be out the door by two so that we could travel two hours to arrive at the airport at four o'clock for check in. Just thinking about when we would have to go to bed and even if we could fall sleep for few hours was stressful. We did consider staying overnight closer to the airport, but decided not to.

This kind of travel, or even a modification of this schedule, can be trying for the person who is diabetic. I cannot stress the importance of eating meals as close to the same time every day. Our very early flight did not pose a problem for me because I had prepared a breakfast wrap made of peanut butter and granny smith apple slices for myself and one for my husband. I forced myself to eat a banana too. I ate the wrap around three thirty in the morning, which provided me with slow-burning carbohydrates and proteins that would last for several hours. My diabetic husband chose not to eat anything, claiming, "It's just too early!" We arrived in Mexico at about twelve thirty, and had to wait for our family members to arrive at different times. My husband started to crash; I had to get some food into him. This probably would not have happened if we'd had time to grab a bite during our one-and-a-half-hour layover in Miami. However, there hadn't been time. We'd had to take a shuttle to another terminal, making a connecting flight with very little time to spare until boarding. My husband drank a Coke from Miami to Cancun. Probably not the best thing. Airlines don't provide snacks to their clients anymore. Unless you go first class, you must bring your own food with you. This is something I have learned to do. I knew our day would be very long, and we wouldn't always be able to depend on having time to eat. This was a very valuable lesson for my husband.

However, "we can all fit into this category" (84). Meaning the health care professional is no exception. A full appointment schedule on top of pressing everyday responsibilities can leave the busy professional with very little time for himself or herself. This is particularly true if the professional has young children with activities of their own. There are meals to plan and shop for and prepare, laundry to wash, sporting events that require transportation and sometimes participation. All of this leaves professionals with very little time to exercise, let alone eat healthfully. It is convenient to grab a burger en route to practice or on the way home. Did I mention that children often need help with homework? After bath time there is story time. I cannot tell you how many times I have fallen asleep while my seven-year-old practiced reading to me!

Most of us can find ways to handle our stresses on a day-to-day, week-to-week basis. Minivacations or longer vacations planned into our work schedules can do wonders to lift the spirit (85). I heard a blip on the radio today stating that patients want doctors to prescribe vacation time for them because, after just one week on holiday, many patients stated they felt refreshed and more energized. I have had what I consider a good work schedule. It is four ten-hour days with a floating day off so that, once a month, I had a four-day weekend. This works great as long as the schedule does not get changed! This can work if there is adequate staff. Everyone needs to find a way to work more efficiently, more productively, and with more energy. Having a minivacation every month may be the answer. The February 2015 issue of *Outside* magazine states that "Ayurvedic hospitals and spas treat 90-year-old farmers with arthritis and stressed-out Western execs who fly in on private jets for monthlong treatments" (86). These clients, while on a month-long vacation, must abide by the strict Ayurvedic principles. I would probably not have trouble adhering to these practices, especially when staying for a month at Somatheeram

Ayurvedic Health Resort, which sits in a tropical garden overlooking the Arabian Sea (87).

What exactly is the ideal diet for the professional? I think the ideal diet should be one that provides energy throughout the day with enough reserve energy for family time after work and for exercise. I was a busy professional while my kids were growing up. Several of my children played on competitive soccer teams. I tried to plan meals and snacks ahead of time. As for exercise, one of the practice fields was surrounded by a five-mile track. While the kids were practicing soccer drills, I pushed the baby in the stroller on a five-mile hike. So you see, there are many ways of getting time for ourselves that involve exercise.

The following diet plan is as ideal as we can get. It provides foods to nourish the body and keep it energized. You may not be able to follow it as recommended. However, adopting some of the helpful suggestions may go a long way to helping you look and feel energized and healthy.

The Ideal Diet

The ideal diet is very good for weight loss and maintenance, provided we pay attention to quantities so we don't overeat. It is well balanced; it is a rotation diet, which means it is good for food allergies; it is high in fiber from whole grains and vegetables; it is low in fat; and it contains good-quality protein. The ideal diet looks like this:

Early Morning:

- one or two pieces of fruit

Breakfast:

- starch (a cereal grain or potatoes)

Midmorning snack:

- fruit

Lunch:

- protein
- green vegetables
- other vegetables

Midafternoon snack:

- vegetable or fruit

Dinner:

- starch or protein
- vegetable

Evening snack:

- vegetable or fruit, if needed

Water is important. You should consume eight to ten glasses of pure water—not chlorinated—throughout the day, especially about one hour before meals. A good multiple vitamin and mineral supplement along with water and fiber and more filling, low-calorie foods will help decrease the appetite. "Water and fiber are the two most useful and inexpensive nutrients for weight reduction and maintenance. They will also support good colon function, which helps to detoxify the body and reduces food cravings" (88).

Healthful eating is manageable and should not be a daunting task. Making a menu plan for the week and shopping accordingly helps to ensure that fresh, whole food ingredients are readily available, and this plan also reduces food waste. Keep snacks handy in the refrigerator such as low-fat cheese sticks, carrots, celery, broccoli, grapes, apples, and oranges. This is a great way to eat healthfully! Hard-boiled eggs are another way of getting protein in the diet, too, and can be prepared ahead of time.

If we eat healthfully and get appropriate exercise, adequate sleep, and time for relaxation, then the stresses of job and lifestyle will be in balance, and we can look forward to healthful living.

Concluding Thoughts

I wrote this book to help people realize the devastating effects stress has on the body. By understanding what triggers our stress, we can become aware of our stressors and hopefully do something about them.

This book shows that, from a historical perspective, diet and exercise go hand in hand and have for decades. Life is not over at sixty-two! That's not the time to succumb to chronic ailments that will eventually lead to premature death. Our bodies, created by the divine author of life, are made to heal themselves given the right kind of nutrients.

Exercise is also vitally important for health. Too little or too much equally can cause harm. It is doubtful that most people would have to worry about too much exercise. A brisk walk in the early morning or evening is something most people can do. The important thing is to *move your body every day!* I enjoy yoga stretches as well as a brisk two- to three-mile walk. In the summer, I prefer swimming. I particularly enjoyed training for a 5K race using the program, From Couch to 5K. I loved sweating because it is a natural way for the body to rid itself of toxins. I will caution, though, excessive sweating can drain sodium reserves from the body. Sodium can be replaced through the consumption of organic foods such as okra, papaya, pears, pineapple, pumpkin, raspberries, brown rice, strawberries, and watermelon, to name a few

We develop diseases by living the kind of lifestyle that contributes to that disease. By changing the lifestyle, particularly a sedentary one, we have the opportunity to live a better life. I would be remiss if I did not discuss diet. While coffee and doughnuts may be a treat once in a while, daily consumption of such foods only brings about aches and pains. We find ourselves therefore reaching for the medicine cabinet to relieve our symptoms. And every doctor knows, as Dr. Bernard Jensen aptly states, "symptom suppression through drugs will not bring better health tomorrow."

Better health comes from eating the right kind of nutrients, getting adequate exercise and sleep, and spending time at leisurely pursuits. Don't put off that vacation!

For a better tomorrow, live each day in harmony and balance.

Live, love, and above all dance ...

Yours in health,

Stephanie Jack, PhD

Notes

1. Center for Science in the Public Interest, Washington, DC.
2. J. Challem, B. Berkson, and M. Smith, *Syndrome X: The Complete Nutrition Program to Prevent and Reverse Insulin Resistance* (New York: John Wiley and Sons, 2000), 38.
3. A Colbain, *Food and Our Bones* (New York: Penguin Putnam, 1998), 32.
4. Ibid, 32.
5. J. Challem, B. Berkson, and M. Smith, *Syndrome X: The Complete Nutrition Program to Prevent and Reverse Insulin Resistance* (New York: John Wiley and Sons, 2000).
6. C. Pfeiffer, *Nutrition and Mental Illness and Orthomolecular Approach to Balancing Body Chemistry* (Rochester: Healing Arts Press, 1987), 4.
7. J. Challem, B. Berkson, and M. Smith, *Syndrome X: The Complete Nutrition Program to Prevent and Reverse Insulin Resistance* (New York: John Wiley and Sons, 2000), 38.
8. S. Collins, RN, North Country Community Health Center, Flagstaff, AZ.
9. E. Haas, *Staying Healthy with Nutrition: The Complete Guide to Diet and Nutritional Medicine* (Berkley: Celestial Arts, 1992), 850.
10. J. Challem, B. Berkson, and M. Smith, *Syndrome X: The Complete Nutrition Program to Prevent and Reverse Insulin Resistance* (New York: John Wiley and Sons, 2000), 40.
11. A. Colbin, *Food and Our Bones*, 30.
12. Ibid, 30.
13. S. Sinatra, *Heart Sense for Women: Your Plan for Natural Prevention and Treatment* (Washington, DC: Lifeline Press, 2000), 246.
14. Bernard Jensen, *Arthritis, Rheumatism, and Osteoporosis: An Effective Program for Correction through Nutrition* (Escondido: Bernard Jensen, 1986), 116.
15. Ibid, 116.
16. B. Jensen, and M. Anderson, *Empty Harvest* (New York: Avery Penguin Putnam, 1990), vii.
17. Ibid, vii.

18. Ibid, 46.
22. http://www.webmd.com 1/28/2015 Goldberg 2014.
23. J. McClintock, *Basic Anatomy and Physiology of the Human Body* (USA, John Wiley and Sons 1975), 553.
24. Ibid.
25. http://www.diabetes.org/living with diabetes/complications'/ mental-health/stress.html.
26. http://www.stress.org/stress-effects 1/24/11.
27. http://www.diabetes.org/livingwith-diabetes/complications/mental-health/stress.html.
28. National Institute of health, *The Impact of Psychological Stress on Wound Healing: Methods and Mechanisms,* Retrieved January 24, 2015.
29. J. Smythies, *Every Person's Guide to Antioxidants* (New Brunswick, New Jersey, London: Rutgers University Press, 1998), 81.
30. Ibid.
31. J. Williams, *Prolonging Health* (Charlottesville: Hampton Roads Publishing Company, 2003), 4.
32. B. Jensen, Arthritis, *Rheumatism, and Osteoporosis: An Effective Program for Correction Through Nutrition* (Escondido: Bernard Jensen, 1986), Introduction.
33. Ibid, Introduction.
34. Ibid, Introduction.
35. Ibid, 1–3.
36. Ibid.
37. Ibid, 8.
38. Ibid, 8.
39. Ibid, 8.
40. Ibid, 11–12.
41 Ibid, 13.
42. Ibid, 14.
43. Ibid, 116.
44. Ibid, 5.
45. Ibid, 5.
46. Ibid, 5.
47. Ibid, 6.
48. Ibid, 146–148.

49. P. Holford, *The Optimum Nutrition Bible* (Berkeley: The Crossing Press, 1999), 53.

50. E. Haas, *Staying Healthy Through Nutrition: the Complete Guide to Diet and Nutritional Medicine* (Berkeley: Celestial Arts, 1992), 434.

51. Ibid, 437.

52. P. Holford, *The Optimum Nutrition Bible* (Berkeley: The Crossing Press, 1999), 53.

53. B. Jensen and M. Anderson, *Empty Harvest* (New York: Avery Penguin Putnam, 1990), 7.

54. Ibid, 7.

55. Ibid, 13.

56. L. Medford, *Why Do I Need Whole Food Supplements* (OK: LDN Publishing, 1949), 34.

57. J. Robert Hatherill, *Eat to Beat Cancer* (New York: Renaissance Books/ St. Martin's Press, 1998), 17.

58. Ibid, 17.

59. Ibid, 18.

60. Ibid, xiv.

61. Ibid, 91.

62. Ibid, 86.

63. L. Medford, *Why Do I Need Whole Food Supplements* (OK: LDN Publishing, 1949), 91–92.

64. Ibid, 93.

65. Ibid, 96.

66. J. Challem, B. Berkson, and M. Smith, *Syndrome X: The Complete Nutrition Program to Prevent and Reverse Insulin Resistance* (New York: John Wiley and Sons, 2000), 141.

67. Ibid, 1.

68. J. Williams, *Prolonging Health* (Charlottesville: Hampton Roads Publishing Company 2003), 22.

69. Men's Journal, Jan-Feb 2015, p. 98

70. J. Williams, *Prolonging Health* (Charlottesville: Hampton Roads Publishing Company 2003), 221.

71. V, Lad, *The Complete Book of Ayurvedic Home Remedies* (New York: Three Rivers Press, 1998), 60.

72. B. Jensen, *Arthritis, Rheumatism and Osteoporosis: An Effective Program for Correction Through Nutrition* (Escondido: Bernard Jensen, 1986), 22.

73. Ibid, 31.
74. J. Challem, B. Berkson, and M. Smith, *Syndrome X: The Complete Nutrition Program to Prevent and Reverse Insulin Resistance* (New York: John Wiley and Sons, 2000), 146.
75. Ibid, 146.
76. Ibid, 147.
77. Ibid, 150.
78. A. Chips, *Killing Your Cancer Without Killing Yourself* (Kill Devil Hills: Transpersonal Publishing, 2006), 117.
79. Ibid, 117.
80. Ibid, 118.
81. W. Price, *Nutrition and Physical Degeneration, 6ᵗʰ Edition* (La Mesa: Price Pottenger Nutrition Foundation, 2004), 24.
82. Ibid, 29.
83. J. Challem, B. Berkson, and M. Smith, *Syndrome X: The Complete Nutrition Program to Prevent and Reverse Insulin Resistance* (New York: John Wiley and Sons, 2000), 151–152.
84. E. Haas, *Staying Healthy with Nutrition: the Complete Guide to Diet and Nutritional Medicine* (Berkeley: Celestial Arts, 1992), 796.
85. Ibid, 796.
86. Outside Magazine, February 2015, p.60.
87. Ibid, 67.
88. E. Haas, *Staying Healthy with Nutrition: the Complete Guide to Diet and Nutritional Medicine* (Berkeley: Celestial Arts, 1992), 850.

Index

www.ingramcontent.com/pod-product-compliance
Lightning Source LLC
Chambersburg PA
CBHW030521290526
45786CB00004B/1564